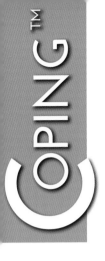

COPING WITH
SEXUALLY TRANSMITTED
DISEASES

Jacqueline Parrish

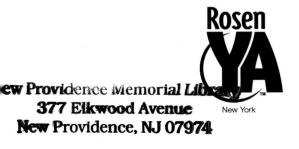

Rosen
YA™

New York

To all of the sexual health activists who have made it their work to end the negative stigma associated with having an STD and for providing educational information to empower people through their diagnosis

Published in 2020 by The Rosen Publishing Group, Inc.
29 East 21st Street, New York, NY 10010

Copyright © 2020 by The Rosen Publishing Group, Inc.

First Edition

B&T 38.47 5/21

Library of Congress Cataloging-in-Publication Data

Names: Parrish, Jacqueline, author.
Title: Coping with sexually transmitted diseases / Jacqueline Parrish.
Description: First edition. | New York : Rosen Publishing, 2020. | Series: Coping |
Audience: Grades 7–12. | Includes bibliographical references and index.
Identifiers: LCCN 2019013376| ISBN 9781725341296 (library bound) |
ISBN 9781725341289 (pbk.)
Subjects: LCSH: Sexually transmitted diseases—Juvenile literature.
Classification: LCC RC200.25 .P37 2020 | DDC 616.95—dc23
LC record available at https://lccn.loc.gov/2019013376

Manufactured in China

On the cover: Being diagnosed with an STD can make you feel confused and alone. The most important thing you can do is thoroughly educate yourself about your condition. It is possible to live a happy life and enjoy healthy sexual relationships.

DISCLAIMER: Some of the images in this book illustrate individuals who are models. The depictions do not imply actual situations or events.

CONTENTS

INTRODUCTION

The United States has become the country with the highest rate of sexually transmitted diseases (STDs) in the industrialized world, according to David Harvey, executive director of the National Coalition of STD Directors (NCSD). The burden of STDs is also a global problem as there are roughly 357.4 million new infections—about one million cases per day— according to the World Health Organization (WHO). There are also roughly 500 million people around the world who have herpes and an estimated 290 million women who have human papillomavirus (HPV). According to a February 2019 article on WHO.int, "More than 1 million sexually transmitted infections (STIs) are acquired every day worldwide. Each year, there are an estimated 357 million new infections with 1 of 4 STIs: chlamydia, gonorrhea, syphilis and trichomoniasis."

Teenagers represent the highest number of STD cases per year, and per the Centers for Disease Control and Prevention (CDC), roughly half of the 19.7 million cases are people between the ages of fifteen and twenty-four. In the book *Sexually Transmitted Diseases: Your Questions Answered*, author Paul Quinn states, "Regardless of advances in science, technology, or pharmaceuticals, an estimated 19.7 million STDs are diagnosed each year in the United States alone.

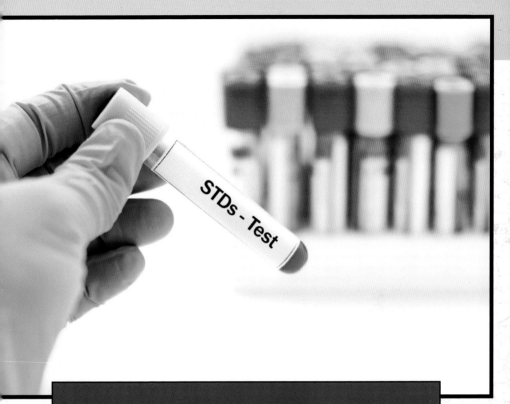

If you're sexually active, take control of your sexual health by getting an STD test. STD tests are often quick, confidential, and painless and can be administered free of charge.

This translates, then, to mean that approximately 1 out of 4 teens will contract an STD."

Increases in STD occurrences can be attributed to many factors, such as the rise in sexual activity among teenagers and the ways in which social media makes it easy to explore sexuality through research, sexting, and/or pornography. It can also be attributed to a lack of prevention and treatment. According to Alexandra Sifferlin's *Time* article, "Only 22 states and the District of Columbia mandate both sex education and HIV [human immunodeficiency virus] education, and many schools provide an abstinence-only curriculum. Sex-education classes often focus largely on preventing unintended pregnancies and less on preventing infections." Finally, the increase in STD occurrences can be attributed to teens not knowing they are infected and engaging in sexual activities. Some STDs manifest no immediate outward symptoms, which causes carriers to think they are healthy and continue to engage in sexual activity. HIV is one such example of an STD that does not show immediate symptoms. According to "Basic Statistics" on CDC.gov, "An estimated 1.1 million people in the United States had HIV at the end of 2016, the most recent year for which this information is available. Of those people, about 14%, or 1 in 7, did not know they had HIV."

If you have been diagnosed with an STD, it is important to remember that you are not alone. STDs are very common, and studies have shown that those who are sexually active will contract at least one STD during their lifetime. Educate yourself on how to cope with an STD diagnosis and why testing (also known as STD screening) is important if you plan to be sexually active. Discover the many resources that are at your fingertips to guide you through the process of coping with an STD. Find out where you can turn for help, how to get proper treatment, and how to live a healthy lifestyle in the wake of an STD diagnosis.

You're Not Alone

STDs are diseases that are passed from person to person via blood, vaginal fluid, or semen during a vaginal, anal, or oral sexual act or pregnancy and childbirth. CDC.gov notes that you do not have to have sexual intercourse to contract an STD. Herpes and HPV, to name a couple, are spread through skin-to-skin contact.

What Are the Different STDs?

There are a variety of STDs, some with immediate symptoms and others that show up much later. This makes it very important to get tested if you are, or plan to be, sexually active.

Chlamydia, Gonorrhea, and Trichomoniasis

Chlamydia and gonorrhea are bacterial infections that can be easily treated with a prescription antibiotic. Trichomoniasis is a parasitic STD, meaning it lives off another host organism, that is also easily treated with medication. Symptoms can include pain during urination, discharge from the vagina, penis, or anus, and lower belly pain.

Pubic Lice

Pubic lice, also known as "crabs" or "pediculosis pubis," are tiny insects that live in pubic hair. They are spread through sexual contact, and symptoms include itchiness, redness, and irritation in the genital region. Condoms and dental dams do not protect against pubic lice, but it is easily treatable with a medicated cream, shampoo, or lotion that can be purchased over-the-counter at a local pharmacy.

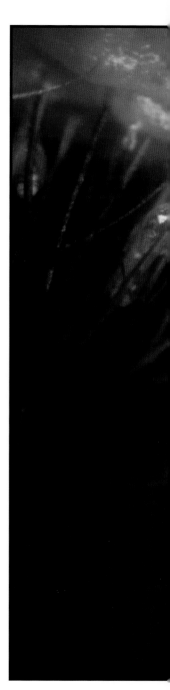

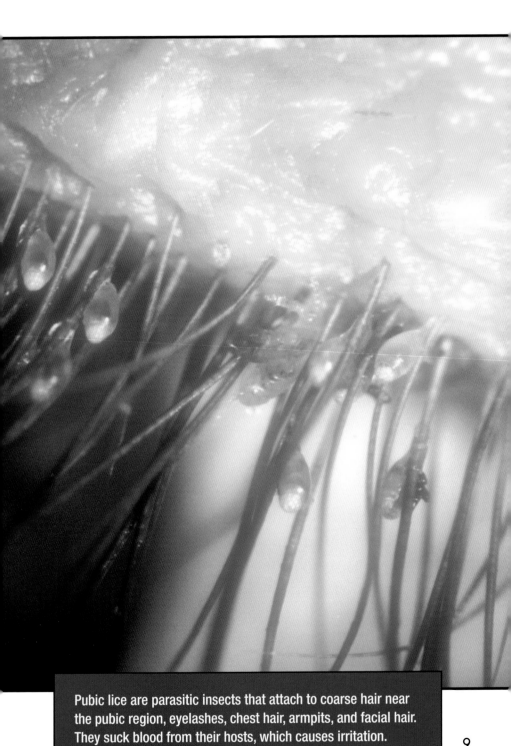

Pubic lice are parasitic insects that attach to coarse hair near the pubic region, eyelashes, chest hair, armpits, and facial hair. They suck blood from their hosts, which causes irritation.

Trichomoniasis

Trichomoniasis is a parasitic STD that manifests almost no symptoms. According to the CDC, trichomoniasis is the most common curable STD. Only 30 percent of people with trichomoniasis experience symptoms, which might include itching and irritation in the genital area, pain during urination, and/or discharge from the penis or vagina. Medication is prescribed for trichomoniasis, and it is suggested that you wait at least one week before engaging in sexual activity.

Syphilis

Syphilis is an STD that is usually accompanied by sores in the genital area. In the first stage of syphilis, the sores are generally painless, are present a few weeks after sexual intercourse, and can disappear without the presence of other symptoms. The second stage of syphilis develops a few weeks after the sores appear. It can include a rash and flu-like symptoms, such as fever, tiredness, muscle aches, and swollen lymph nodes. If caught early, syphilis is easily treated with penicillin. If left untreated, it can be life threatening, eventually affecting the brain, heart, eyes, or nerves.

HPV and Genital Herpes

HPV is a group of viruses that can cause noncancerous warts or cancer of the cervix, throat, mouth, vulva, vagina, penis, and anus. It is the most common STD that affects all genders. Seventy-nine million people in the United States have HPV, and there are roughly fourteen million new cases each year according to Cancer.org. Many doctors compare contracting HPV to catching the common cold since it is so common. The CDC states that more than 90 percent of people who are sexually active will have HPV at least once in their lives.

People who have genital herpes do not know they are infected until they have an outbreak. An outbreak consists of sores in the genital area. Outbreaks can happen when the person is stressed, overly tired, or during sickness. Genital herpes is a viral infection, which means there is no cure, but it can be easily managed with medication that helps prevent or shorten an outbreak. There are two types of genital herpes viruses, herpes simplex virus type 1 (HSV-1) and herpes simplex virus type 2 (HSV-2). Genital herpes is one of the most common STDs, and it is estimated that one out of eight people have the virus in the United States.

The HPV Vaccination

The Food and Drug Administration (FDA) has approved three vaccinations to protect against the types of HPV that cause cervical cancer: Gardasil, Gardasil 9, and Cervarix. The American Cancer Society suggests that boys and girls receive the HPV vaccination Gardasil or Gardasil 9 at eleven or twelve years old, although the vaccination can be given up to age twenty-six. Cervarix can be administered to young girls as early as age nine. According to Cancer.org, "The vaccines work best at this age. Research shows that younger people have a better immune response to the vaccine than those in their late teens and early 20s." The vaccinations have proven to be effective at protecting against new HPV infections.

(continued on page 14)

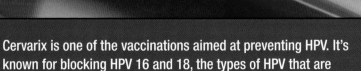

Cervarix is one of the vaccinations aimed at preventing HPV. It's known for blocking HPV 16 and 18, the types of HPV that are responsible for causing 70 percent of cervical cancer cases.

(continued from page 12)

The vaccinations, however, are not effective at treating an already established HPV infection.

On October 5, 2018, the FDA announced that Gardasil 9 is now approved for females and males between the ages of twenty-seven and forty-five. According to the FDA website, Dr. Peter Marks said, "Today's approval represents an important opportunity to help prevent HPV-related diseases and cancers in a broader age range." Due to the overwhelming amount of HPV-related cases per year, creating a vaccination for a broader age group was a top priority. It is estimated that fourteen million people in the United States are diagnosed with HPV every year, and that doesn't include the global epidemic. It is estimated that twelve thousand women are diagnosed with an HPV-related cancer and roughly four thousand women die each year from HPV-related cervical cancer.

Genital herpes is also a global issue because it is estimated that 412 million people universally are also infected with the virus.

HIV/AIDS

HIV is a virus that is contracted through sexual intercourse or sharing a needle with an infected person through drug use or tattooing. The virus attacks the person's immune system, making it harder for the person to fight infections such as the common cold. Due to the mild symptoms of HIV—including fever, headache, and painful ulcers—a person may not know he or she is infected until HIV reaches the stage of AIDS. AIDS (acquired immune deficiency syndrome) develops when a person has had HIV for many years. AIDS is a very serious medical condition that severely weakens a person's immune system and potentially causes death.

Hepatitis B

Hepatitis B can be transmitted through semen and vaginal secretions during sexual intercourse. It can cause cancer and liver failure if left untreated and in some cases, lead to death. Many people with the hepatitis B virus do not know they have it until a blood test is administered. In many cases, patients diagnosed with hepatitis B fully recover if their immune system is strong enough to fight the infection. It is recommended that all newborn babies receive the first dose of the hepatitis B vaccination when they are born. The vaccination is followed up by three to four shots over a period of time.

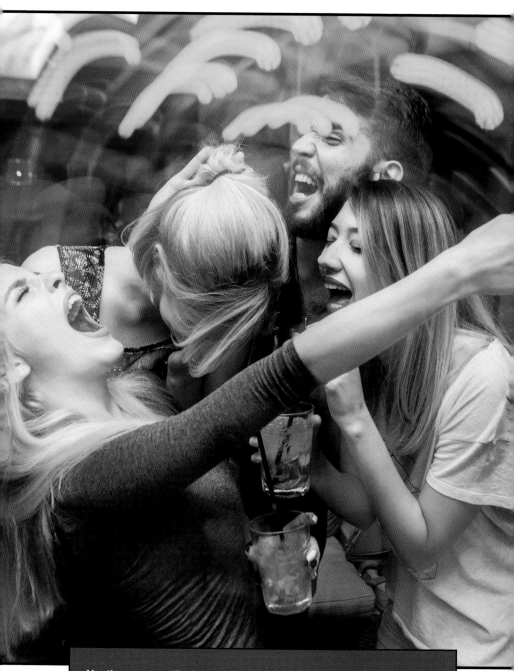

Youth are more likely to be involved in risky sexual behavior, which could lead to the spread of STDs. Young adults account for half of all new STD cases.

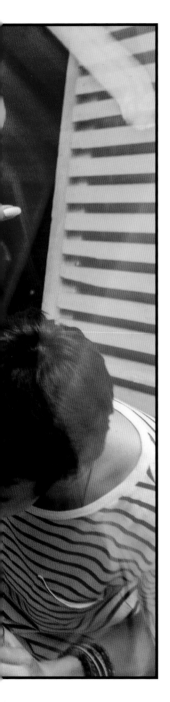

On its website, the WHO states, "The vaccine against hepatitis B has already prevented an estimated 1.3 million deaths from chronic liver disease and cancer."

Risky Sexual Behavior

It is common for young people to engage in risky sexual behavior, whether it's because they feel adventurous or give in to peer pressure. According to the CDC website, 46 percent of young people who had engaged in sexual intercourse during the past three months did not use a condom, and 19 percent had used alcohol or drugs during their last sexual experience. It was also noted that 14 percent of people did not use any protection to prevent pregnancy. An article titled "Sexual Intercourse Among High School Students—29 States and United States Overall, 2005–2015" on the CDC website states, "The

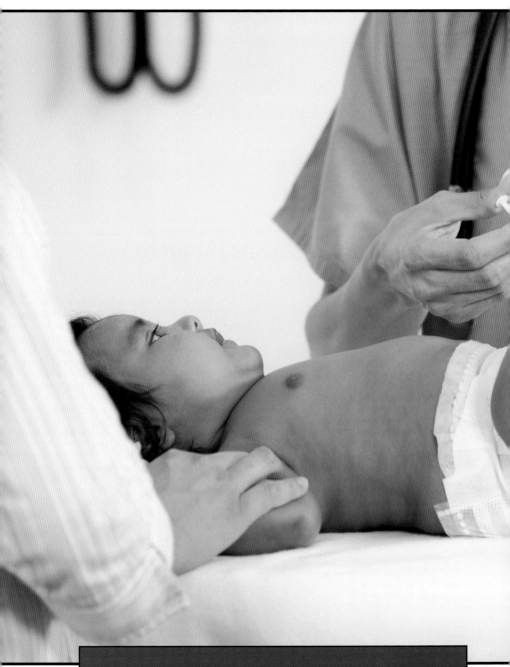

The first dose of the hepatitis B vaccination is given to a newborn within twenty-four hours of birth. The vaccine stimulates the immune system to protect against the virus.

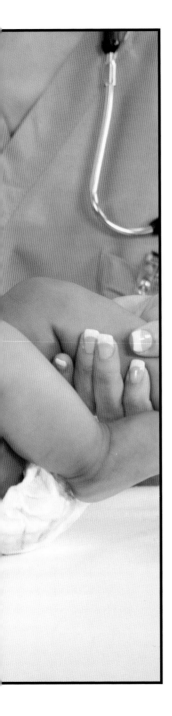

majority of adolescents initiate sexual activity during high school, and the proportion of high school students who have ever had sexual intercourse increases by grade."

The Only Way to Prevent STDs

Abstinence is the surest way to prevent exposure to an STD. Only by refraining from sexual intercourse (vaginal or anal) and oral sex can one truly prevent contracting HIV and STDs, and avoid unwanted pregnancy. It is OK to say no if you aren't comfortable having sex. Sometimes peer pressure is introduced when it comes to having sex. Some teens may feel the need to have sex because their friends are doing it or the person they are dating is pressuring them. Another way to reduce exposure is being mutually monogamous with your partner.

Mutually monogamous means that you have come to an agreement with your sexual partner and have decided to only have sexual contact with each other after being tested for STDs. Avoid mixing alcohol, drugs, and sexual intercourse. Alcohol and drugs increase your likelihood of taking a risk, such as having sexual intercourse without protection or having sexual contact with someone you wouldn't normally have sex with if you were sober. It is estimated that one-quarter of high school aged students have used alcohol or drugs when they were last sexually active. Teenagers who use alcohol or drugs are more likely to risk unprotected sexual intercourse and have multiple sexual partners, which increases the chance of contracting an STD.

Prevention Education

STDs are on the rise despite the abundance of information available regarding STD prevention. Education is key to learning and preventing exposure to STDs and to receiving proper treatment to stay healthy. Keep in mind that comprehensive sexual education doesn't encourage youths to go out and have sex, but it doesn't suggest they can't either. Dr. Elizabeth Boskey wrote the following for a VeryWellHealth.com article:

Comprehensive sex education doesn't encourage kids to have sex. Just like abstinence-only programs, good comprehensive programs teach students that abstinence is the only surefire way to prevent pregnancy and STDs. The difference is that these programs also give students realistic and factual information about the safety of various sexual practices, and how to improve the odds.

Health-care providers can provide essential information regarding your sexual health and offer STD testing and vaccinations for HPV and hepatitis B. However, it isn't always easy to obtain accurate information and patient-specific treatment plans outside of a doctor's office. Author Paul Quinn writes the following in *Sexually Transmitted Diseases: Your Questions Answered*:

Education has been highlighted as a key strategy toward reducing, or eliminating, STDs. In the modern age, the explosion of information available on the Internet has been both a benefit and a hindrance to combatting STDs. The suggestions for care, treatment, or prevention are often vague, doing little to reduce the fear or stigma associated with actual or potential STDs.

If you are thinking about having sexual intercourse or are currently sexually active, there are many ways to educate yourself on STD education and prevention. Abstinence is abstaining from any sexual contact, whether it is sexual intercourse or oral sex. Get tested for STDs before any sexual contact has occurred with a new partner, be mutually monogamous with your partner, educate yourself on proper protection, and do not mix drugs and alcohol with sex, which might increase your chance of taking a risk, such as engaging in sexual activity without a condom or dental dam. All of these activities can help prevent you from contracting an STD.

Myths & FACTS

Myth: You can get an STD by sitting on a public toilet.

Fact: There is no scientific evidence that you can get an STD by sitting on a toilet. The bacteria and viruses that you could get from sexual contact, or skin-to-skin contact, cannot live outside of the body for long.

Myth: You can't get an STD if you have anal or oral sex.

Fact: STDs are contracted through genital contact, semen, and blood. They can also be contracted via oral sex and cause symptoms in the mouth and/or throat. The STDs that can be spread via oral sex include chlamydia, gonorrhea, syphilis, herpes, HPV, HIV, and trichomoniasis.

Myth: I will know if my partner has an STD.

Fact: Many STDs do not show physical symptoms. STDs such as HPV and chlamydia rarely present any symptoms, making it important to get tested if and when you are sexually active.

CHAPTER TWO

Opening Up and Getting Help

Many teens believe they are not at risk for an STD, largely due to a lack of open dialogue regarding sex and its possible results. In a *Time* article, epidemiologist Eloisa Llata states, "Everyone should talk more—and more openly—about STDs in order to raise awareness and reduce stigma." There are many people that you can consider to be a confidant, including a trusted parent or guardian, sibling, extended family member, friend, partner, teacher or school counselor, spiritual leader, therapist, or medical professional.

If you're looking for help beyond those who know you personally, consider reaching out to Planned Parenthood. This nonprofit organization specializes in sexual and reproductive health, and

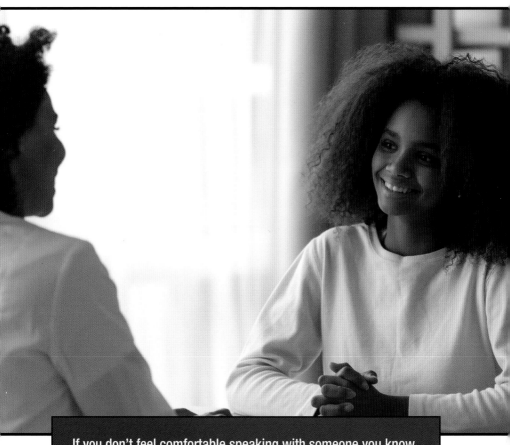

If you don't feel comfortable speaking with someone you know about STDs, there are many confidential resources through Planned Parenthood and your local health department.

offers free and low-cost STD testing. According to PlannedParenthood.org, the organization provides confidential, high-quality reproductive health care for all ages, sexual orientations, and gender identities. Its website also states that you do not need your parent's or guardian's permission to get an STD test and the results will never be released to your parent or guardian.

25

Preparing for the Doctor

The best rule of thumb when seeing a doctor is to be open, honest, and prepared. Before your appointment, create a list of questions you would like to ask to properly educate yourself. You have the right to ask questions about the examination or procedure, which is known as "informed consent."

During the intake portion of your appointment, let your doctor know if you are sexually active and whether it involved vaginal, oral, and/or anal sex. Also mention if you have ever had unprotected sex, in this case or with a former partner(s), and if you've experienced pain or bleeding before, during, or after any sexual activities. During your appointment, your doctor will check your genitals to make sure everything looks healthy. Your testing will be based on your anatomy, including a pelvic exam or Pap smear for those with vaginas and a testicle check for those with penises. If you are transgender, it is important that you find a health-care provider who is familiar with the unique needs and health concerns of transgender people.

If at any time you feel uncomfortable or experience pain during the exam, voice your concern to the doctor or nurse. If you want the health-care professional to stop, it is OK to say "stop" even if the procedure has already begun. Remember, this is your body and you have control over it at all times.

Another option to consider is your local health department. They offer free and low-cost STD testing, which is confidential for patients age twelve and older. Most also offer free HIV tests. The type of test you receive from the health department can vary from location to location. Some health departments offer blood and urine STD tests, while others only offer rapid tests. Some health departments won't screen for all STDs, but most will offer testing for gonorrhea, syphilis, chlamydia, and HIV. If you have any questions, you can always contact your local health department to find out more information.

Colleges and universities will often offer students free and low-cost STD testing. Similar to

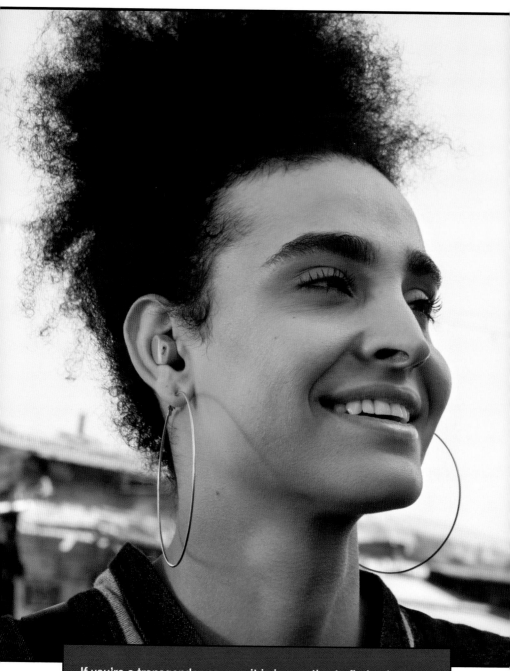

If you're a transgender person, it is imperative to find a doctor or nurse who is sensitive to your health care needs and who will make you feel comfortable during an examination.

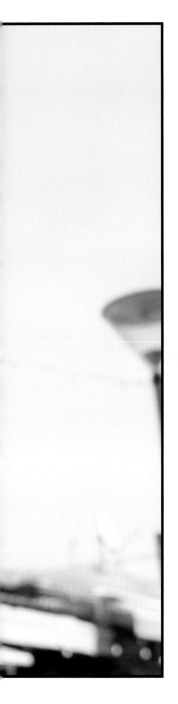

the local health department, these institutions vary in how and what they test for.

Talking to a Parent or Guardian

Talking about sex and STDs can be uncomfortable, even with the closest of relationships. If you choose to open up to a parent or guardian, consider that having a mature discussion could bring you closer. Remember that your parent or guardian was also a teenager at one time, and they might know a lot about sex and STDs that could prove useful in getting the information and/ or testing you need. It might be beneficial to write down all of the questions you want to ask before speaking with them. You can prepare yourself and practice what you will say, or even email or text them if you don't feel comfortable speaking in person. "I know this is awkward, but ..."

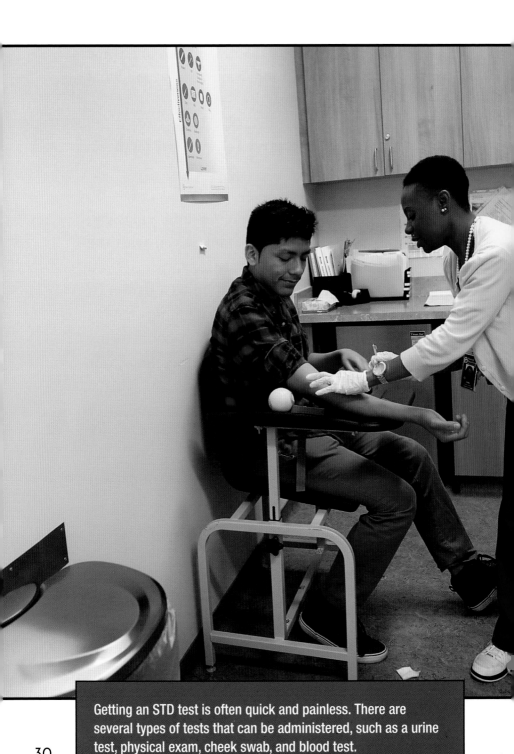

Getting an STD test is often quick and painless. There are several types of tests that can be administered, such as a urine test, physical exam, cheek swab, and blood test.

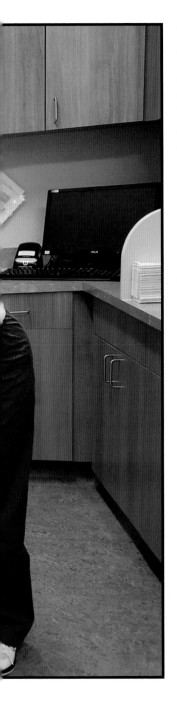

is a great conversation starter that will break the ice during your discussion. Then be open and honest, voicing your concerns and inviting them to ask questions so they can fully understand your situation. According to a January 30, 2014, Planned Parenthood article, "A new nationwide survey released today shows that most parents and teens talk about sex; teens are less comfortable than their parents having these conversations; and parents need to talk more about how their teens can prevent pregnancy and STDs."

If talking to a parent or guardian is not an option, most nonprofit organizations, such as Planned Parenthood, do not need parental consent for you to get tested for STDs. Sexetc.org is a great resource for information regarding STD testing and parental consent laws from state to state. There is also an abundance of information on sex education, living with an STD, and STD testing.

The Difference Between STD and STI

The terms "STD" (sexually transmitted disease) and "STI" (sexually transmitted infection) are synonymous. The popularity of the term "STI" is on the rise due to the stigma associated with the word "disease." The American Sexual Health Association (ASHA) opts to steer away from the word "disease" since a lot of sexual infections do not have any signs or symptoms. In the medical sector, HPV starts out as an infection or an STI and only develops into a disease or STD if it turns into cervical cancer. This is also true of many other STIs, such as chlamydia and gonorrhea, which start out as bacterial infections. Untreated chlamydia and gonorrhea can turn into pelvic inflammatory disease (PID). PID is an infection that affects the female reproductive organs. According to the CDC, the symptoms of PID include bleeding between periods, unusual vaginal discharge, and pain when urinating. If PID is left untreated, it can cause infertility and chronic abdominal pain. Many STIs produce no symptoms, so it is common that people are unaware that they are infected until they develop a disease. That is why getting tested early and often is important.

Talking with Your Partner(s)

The best time to discuss STDs and testing with a new partner is before you engage in sexual activity, regardless of whether your involvement is short- or long-term. Your efforts will show that sexual health is important to you, and having the discussion could strengthen your experience or relationship.

To help you overcome embarrassment, consider jotting down what you want to say ahead of time. Then select a good time and location to speak with your partner so that you won't be interrupted or distracted. Begin the conversation by acknowledging the awkwardness of the topic, and then ask how they would feel about getting tested for STDs. If you have been recently tested or treated for STDs, let them know. Finally, take the time to agree on preferred methods of STD prevention, such as the use of condoms and dental dams.

Actively listen to what your partner has to say and gauge their nonverbal reactions to understand if you are on the same page regarding safe sex and STD testing. If it seems like your partner is hesitant, it could indicate a concern such as the cost of testing, an already-known diagnosis, or a fear of medical offices. Or it could be something entirely different. Keep the conversation going, no matter how awkward, until all of your questions are answered

The stigma surrounding an STD diagnosis is often a reason people don't get tested. Educate yourself and others about STDs to help prevent the negative stigma.

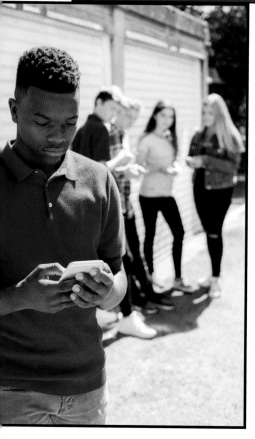

and you are ready to make an informed decision about engaging sexually or not.

Handling the Stigma of an STD

All too frequently there is a stigma associated with having an STD. Many people believe it means that carriers are trashy, dirty, unclean, or promiscuous. This is far from the truth. STDs do not discriminate, and with the rising number of reported cases on the rise in the United States and worldwide, it can be assumed that there are many more carriers who don't know they have an STD. The STD Project takes the consideration of the stigma further by stating the following on TheSTDProject.com: "More importantly, this type of branding does nothing to encourage people to get tested for sexually transmitted infections if they continue to believe, as long as they aren't 'whoring around,' they'll be safe." If you are sexually active, it is your responsibility to get tested.

To help put an end to the stigma associated with having an STD, experts suggest that you educate yourself. The more you know, the more you can educate others about the facts surrounding STDs and put an end to the stigma. STDs are nothing but infections, and since they don't discriminate, anyone can get an STD regardless of whether they are engaging in their first sexual act or their thousandth.

CHAPTER THREE

Where to Turn for Help

A positive diagnosis for an STD can be scary, confusing, and embarrassing, and cause you to feel like the only person in the world who is going through the situation. But you are not alone and you will get through this. Always remember that STDs are very common. According to a February 28, 2019, article on WHO.org:

> *More than 1 million STIs are acquired every day. Each year, there are estimated 357 million new infections with 1 of 4 STIs: chlamydia (131 million), gonorrhea (78 million), syphilis (5.6 million) and trichomoniasis (143 million). More than 500 million people are living with genital HSV (herpes) infection. At any point in time, more than 290 million women*

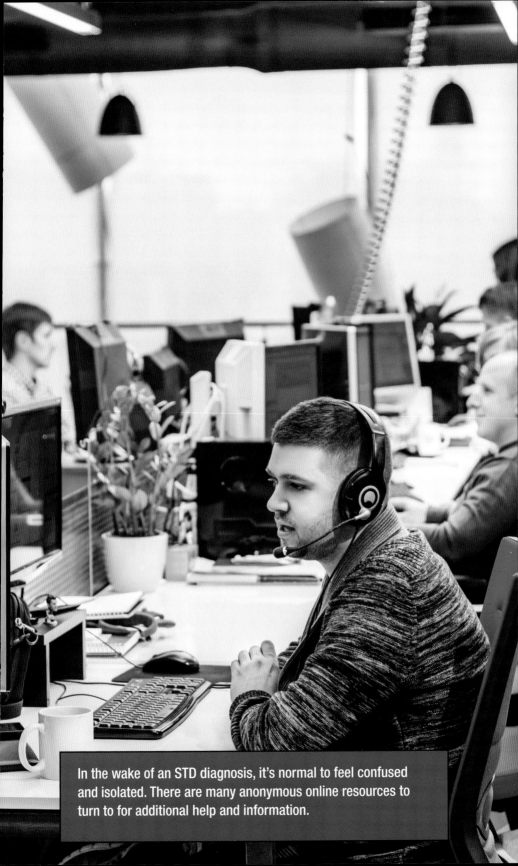

In the wake of an STD diagnosis, it's normal to feel confused and isolated. There are many anonymous online resources to turn to for additional help and information.

have an HPV infection, one of the most common STIs.

According to the WHO, young people between the ages of fifteen and twenty-four had the highest recorded cases of chlamydia. Herpes is another common STD and, according to the CDC, one out of two people between the ages of fourteen and forty-nine are infected with herpes (HSV-1). The rise of STDs in the United States, and globally, means your chances of contracting an STD in your lifetime are pretty high. The statistics suggest that one out of two sexually active individuals will contract an STD by the time they reach age twenty-five. While the statistics are a little scary, they emphasize the fact that contracting an STD is very common for a lot of people.

I Have an STD. Now What?

The first step when receiving a positive diagnosis for an STD is to allow yourself time to process the information. You may be feeling resentment, shame, and/or guilt, which is completely normal. If the diagnosis affects your mental health, reach out to a trusted person in whom to confide. This could be a school counselor, friend, or relative.

Second, be sure to take care of yourself. Schedule an appointment with a doctor who can help you come up with a plan to treat the STD and give your body every opportunity to heal. If you are diagnosed with a bacterial infection, such as chlamydia, gonorrhea, or syphilis, your doctor can prescribe an antibiotic. Once the antibiotic knocks the infection out of your system, you will no longer infect anyone else with the STD. If you are diagnosed with a viral infection, such as HPV or herpes, your doctor can teach you how to manage your symptoms.

The third step in dealing with a positive diagnosis it to notify all past and current sexual partners so they can be tested and treated. Since many STDs present no symptoms, a past partner may be infected and not know. Although this is often the hardest step for most people, it is one of the most important things you can do. Tracy Clark-Flory writes the following in an article in *Elle*:

> *Lots of infections, including chlamydia, can have zero symptoms and still cause a lot of problems—especially in the long term with fertility. Your past partner, if they don't know that they're at risk for infection, might*

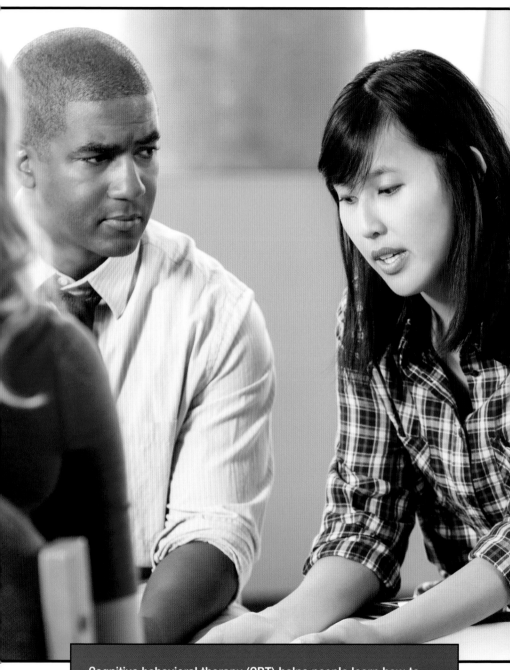

Cognitive behavioral therapy (CBT) helps people learn how to process their environment and cope with everyday stressors, such as being diagnosed and living with an STD.

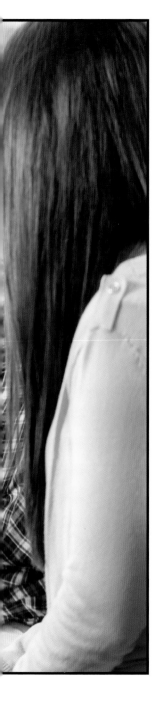

not be protecting themselves in the way that they would if they knew they were at risk.

Talk with a Professional

If being diagnosed with an STD is negatively affecting your life, it might be time to talk with a counselor, therapist, or health-care professional. The information you tell them will always be confidential. These professionals can provide you with unbiased support to help you process and understand the diagnosis, learn ways of coping with it more effectively, and help you set a positive outlook for the future. They can also talk with you about how to practice safe sex to avoid spreading the infection and avoid risky sexual behavior when moving forward.

Mary Elizabeth Dallas notes the following in her Consumer HealthDay article: "Behavioral counseling can reduce the odds of developing a sexually transmitted infection and encourage safe-sex practices, the experts concluded after reviewing previously published studies." One such method is cognitive behavioral therapy (CBT), which is a form of talk therapy that helps you identify and challenge negative thoughts, so you can work through them successfully. It is performed under the direction of a therapist who uses CBT to tackle specific problems and put a focus on goal-oriented approaches. During your CBT sessions, your therapist might encourage "homework" such as specific reading assignments and extracurricular activities. Your therapist may then encourage you to apply what you are learning to your everyday life.

Talking to a health-care provider, such as a doctor or nurse, can also be beneficial in the wake of an STD diagnosis. Your health-care provider can steer

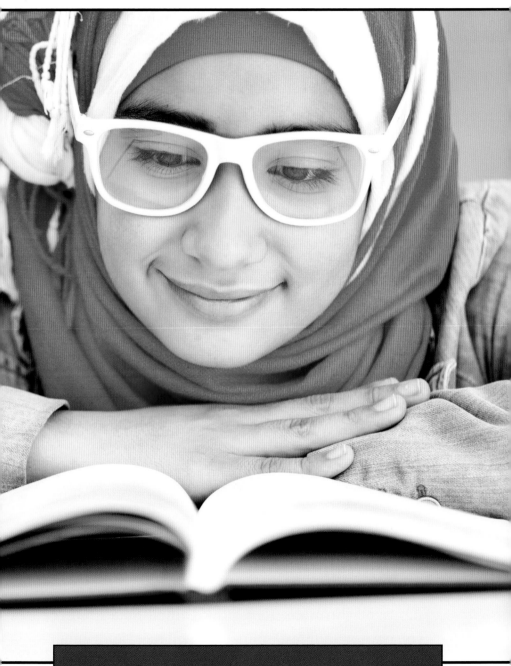

Research suggests that homework in combination with talk therapy increases the overall effectiveness of therapy and leads to improved mental health.

you in the right direction with proper medication and how to take care of your physical health. Bacterial STDs such as chlamydia, gonorrhea, and syphilis are treatable with antibiotics. Your doctor will prescribe the proper antibiotic for the condition and let you know how long to take it for effectiveness. Keep in mind that you will need to follow the instructions to completion in order for the medication to successfully fight off the infection. Viral STDs, such as HPV, herpes, and HIV, are not curable but can be easily treated with medication to reduce the risk of passing the infection on to your partner(s).

Get Tested with Online Support

The stigma associated with STDs can leave you feeling isolated and may cause you to want to turn to help from strangers who do not know you or your situation. STDAware.com is a great online resource for anonymity. From the privacy of your home, you can select an online STD test for chlamydia, gonorrhea, hepatitis A, hepatitis B, hepatitis C, herpes 1, herpes 2, HIV, and syphilis. You can also select a preferred testing site from more than four thousand locations across the United States. Once you pay for your test online, you will receive an email with your lab information to take to your location

I Have an Incurable STD. How Will It Affect My Future?

You might have many emotions after being diagnosed with an STD, especially regarding the future of relationships and sex. Don't limit yourself when it comes to dating but be prepared to bring up the subject when the time arrives. If you are educated and confident about the topic at hand, the conversation may not be as hard as you imagined. There are STD-friendly dating websites, such as Positive Singles (PositiveSingles.com) and Dating Positive (DatingPositives.com) for people with herpes and other STDs. It may be more comfortable for you to find someone who understands and has gone through the same experience you have. The right time to have the conversation with a new partner is different for every dater. Some people prefer to wait and get to know the person before talking about their STD and some people jump right in. It is important to communicate with your partner before any sexual contact to avoid spreading STDs. If the conversation about having an STD is something

(continued on the next page)

(continued from the previous page)

that frightens you, which is completely normal due to the fear of rejection, practice what you will say to the other person. Let your partner know the facts about your STD. Allow your partner to process the information and listen to what they have to say as well. If they aren't supportive and understanding it is time to reevaluate the relationship. There are plenty of fish in the sea. If you find that your diagnosis is negatively affecting your mental health, there is a website called the Trevor Project that is open 24/7 for people who are facing a crisis or are suicidal and need someone to talk to.

of choice. This website can also help you with your STD diagnosis, STD resources, and connecting you to people who can help.

Avoid Negative Self-Talk

It's easy to go down a negative path when you are diagnosed with an STD, but once you realize you aren't alone in the struggle, you can start to pick yourself up again, whether you are feeling scared or uncertain about your future or the diagnosis is

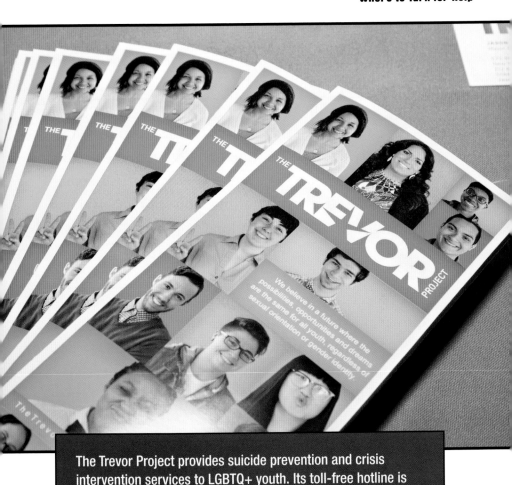

The Trevor Project provides suicide prevention and crisis intervention services to LGBTQ+ youth. Its toll-free hotline is staffed by trained counselors and is completely confidential.

upsetting. It is important to avoid negative self-talk. According to Dr. Ben Martin for PsychCentral in an article dated October 8, 2018, "Self-talk is often skewed towards the negative, and sometimes it's just plain wrong. If you are experiencing depression, it is particularly likely that you interpret things negatively. That's why it's useful to keep an eye on the things you tell yourself, and challenge some of the negative aspects of your thinking."

Allow yourself to react to the diagnosis and grieve the results. Do not shame yourself. You can contract an STD even if it is your first sexual experience. The worst thing you can do is beat yourself up over the situation. Accept the diagnosis and try to move forward in a positive way. It is natural for your mind to wander to the "what-ifs," and that is usually where negative self-talk comes into play. Put your diagnosis into perspective and ask yourself if your thoughts toward the STD are factual. Your mind might automatically jump to a negative conclusion about the STD so it is imperative that you begin to educate yourself.

In order to move forward, you will need to focus on goal-driven thinking. What can you learn from the situation and how can you move forward? If you recognize your negative self-talk you can challenge yourself to look at things in a different light. Sometimes practice makes perfect, and it might be something you need to work at on a daily basis. According to Martin, "With practice, you can learn to notice your own negative self-talk as it happens, and consciously choose to think about the situation in a more realistic and helpful way."

10 Great Questions to Ask a Specialist

1. Can I still have children if I have an STD?

2. Are there ways to prevent my partner or partners from becoming infected?

3. When should my partner or partners be tested?

4. When should I start taking my medication (if needed)?

5. How will this diagnosis affect my daily life in the short and long term?

6. How often should I be tested for STDs?

7. Going forward, how can I prevent the spread of infection?

8. Do any of these tests have a false reading?

9. Should I be retested after my treatment is complete (for bacterial infections)?

10. Are there any resources available to educate myself on my diagnosis?

CHAPTER FOUR

Coping with a Positive STD Diagnosis

The future looks bright for the fight against STDs. Barbara Woolsey's article for Thrillist talks about the future of STD treatment. It notes that HPV is one of the most common STDs and is responsible for more than thirty thousand new cases of cancer each year. There are an estimated eighty million people who are infected with the HPV virus. However, most infections will disappear within two years without detection. HPV is responsible for almost all cervical and anal cancer cases. The introduction of an HPV vaccination has reduced the prevalence of the infection in females. Within six years of introducing a vaccine, there has been an overall decrease in HPV cases by 64 percent in females who are between the ages of fourteen and nineteen. Also, there has been a 34 percent decrease in females aged twenty to twenty-four.

Pre-exposure prophylaxis (PrEP) is a pill that is effective at preventing HIV. According to the CDC, if HIV-negative people take the pill once a day, the chances of contracting HIV decrease by more than 90 percent. PrEP is often given to people who are at a higher risk of developing HIV, such as those with HIV-positive partners. It is recommended that you combine PrEP with condom use because PrEP does not provide protection against other STDs. In combination with condoms, PrEP is highly effective against the spread of HIV.

PPCM, also known as polyphenylene carboxymethylene, is a powerful gel that prevents HIV, herpes, HPV, and even pregnancy. It is in preclinical trials but is expected to also block chlamydia and gonorrhea. Barbara Woolsey, for Thrillist, states, "It's a highly charged polymer that's being developed to block viruses from attaching to host cells that should be available by 2022."

Tenofovir rings are vaginal rings that combine both birth control hormones and HIV prevention. While not yet on the market, the company is looking at developing a dissolving

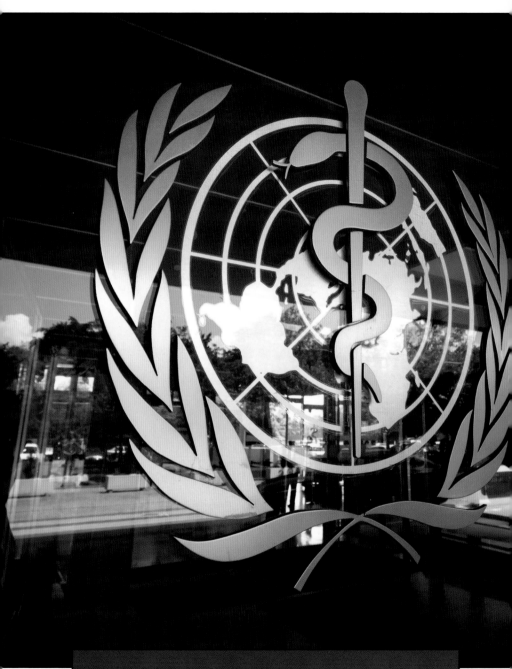

The World Health Organization (WHO) specializes in promoting health, improving access to medicine and other health products worldwide, and detecting and responding to health crises.

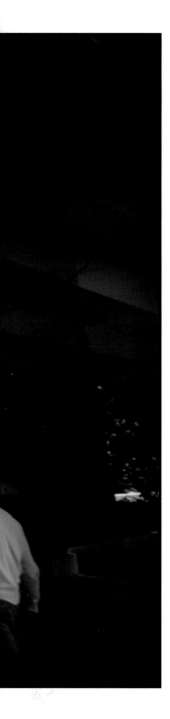

vaginal pill and a gel. The vaginal rings would contain Tenofovir, which is on the market for patients who are HIV-positive. Tenofovir does not cure HIV but lowers the chances of developing AIDS. If used in combination with condoms, it also lowers the chance of spreading HIV to other people.

Hydrogel condoms are the future of condoms and the closest thing to feeling like you aren't wearing a condom at all. Hydrogel is water-based so it feels more like skin than latex condoms. This is important as it is estimated that four out of every ten teenagers ditch condom use because of the sensation, and the number one reason people don't use condoms is because they don't like the way they feel. Experts agree that condoms are the next best thing to abstinence in preventing the spread of STDs, so it makes sense to create a condom that feels like human skin. Hydrogel is self-lubricating,

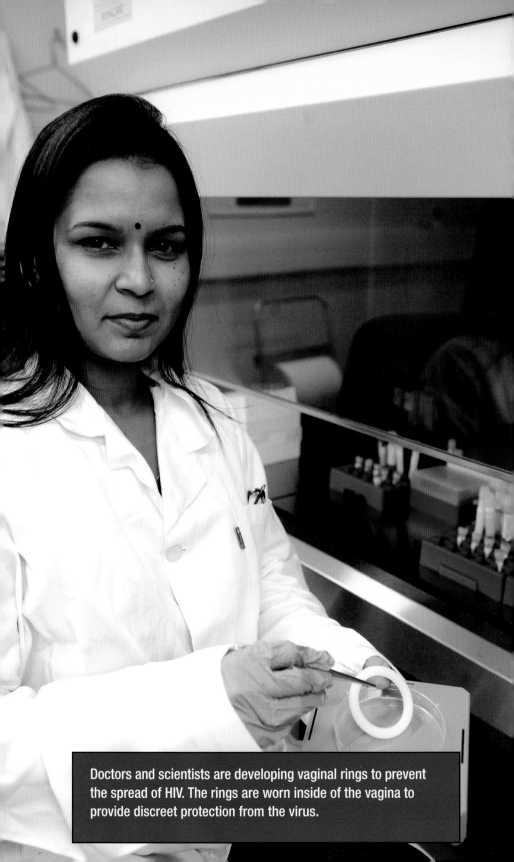

Doctors and scientists are developing vaginal rings to prevent the spread of HIV. The rings are worn inside of the vagina to provide discreet protection from the virus.

helping to prevent breakage, which spreads bacteria, viruses, and sperm. It is also odorless and tasteless, which is especially appealing to those engaged in sexual activities.

A Fresh Perspective

If you have been diagnosed with an STD, it is normal to want to hold someone accountable, especially if you have been diagnosed with an incurable STD. But, you have to learn to redirect the anger you might feel into something positive. Your STD diagnosis does not define who you are as a person. Contracting an STD does not make you "dirty." It is merely an outcome from an experience, and it should not change your perspective of who you are and what you have to contribute to your community.

Practicing Safe Sex

Safe sex means that you actively take steps to prevent the spread of infection to your partner(s). If you have a bacteria-based STD, you will have to take prescribed medication to manage your symptoms and practice safe sex to prevent the spread of disease to current and future partners. If you have a viral-based STD, you will have to practice safe sex for the rest of your life since these infections are not curable.

One of the best ways to practice safe sex is with the use of a condom or dental dam. Keep in mind that a condom does not prevent all STDs. For example, if a condom is used correctly, it can almost fully protect against the spread of HIV. HPV, one of the most common STDs, however, can be found on areas of the body that are not covered by a condom, such a male's scrotum, and can still be spread. While condoms do lower the risk of contracting and spreading HPV, the risk is still there.

Continue to Build Your Support System

As you continue to process your diagnosis, keep the conversation and support going. Talk with an individual or a group of people who understand what you are going through. The STD Project is a great place to start if you are looking to connect with others in a similar situation. You can find support groups by the type of STD you have, such as HIV, herpes, or HPV. There are support groups in the US, Canada, Australia, and the UK, as well as international directories. You can search for support groups depending on your location and get a comprehensive description of the group as well as its contact information. Also, STD Aware has an online resource center that lists online and offline support groups for people infected with herpes, HIV, chlamydia, and syphilis.

Your friends can become a wonderful support group. After all, they are your chosen family. Those you decide to confide in should be loving and supportive. Avoid those who seem insensitive or indifferent, as they will only contribute to the stigma that surrounds STDs. No real friend will put you down for a real-life situation. Do not let their harsh words or judgment impact your self-worth. Do not let your STD diagnosis ruin you; instead allow it to make you a stronger person. Opt for those who prove to be real friends, who build you up, help you out, and support your efforts to claim a healthy future. You may even find that they are going through something similar and can use your help to cope.

Can a Treated STD Rear Its Ugly Head Again?

Once you have been treated for an STD, you might wonder if it can come back. It is very important that you finish all of your medication and take the medication correctly if you are diagnosed with a bacterial STD. Antibiotics require you to take the full amount prescribed, even if you show signs of improvement. Make sure to finish all of

Advancements in HIV Treatment

As of 2019, a cure for HIV has not been found. However, there have been advancements in treatment options. People who are diagnosed as HIV-positive are now living longer lives thanks to advancements in treatment medication. In 1991, basketball superstar Magic Johnson was diagnosed with HIV. At that time, contracting HIV was thought to be a death sentence and a disease that only gay men contracted. Johnson was the first heterosexual public figure to announce his diagnosis. Although the virus ultimately ended his basketball career in 1995, Johnson remains healthy today thanks to following his doctors' orders and taking advanced medications.

One such advancement is antiretroviral therapy (ART). It combines drugs that affect the way the virus is spread. ART is not a cure for HIV, but it helps the virus from reproducing in the bloodstream. HIV is measured by the amount of the virus that is in the patient's bloodstream. ART is administered to get the viral amount in the bloodstream low enough that the blood tests can't detect the virus in the patient. There is hope for a cure in 2020

(continued on page 60)

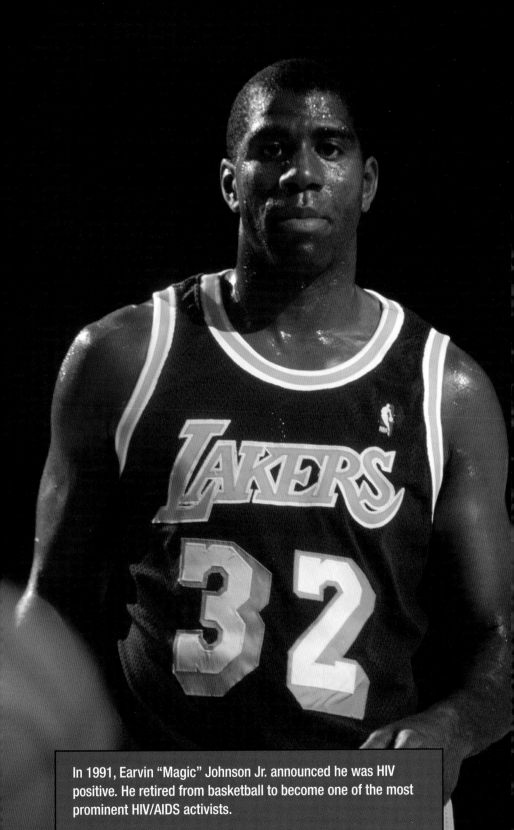

In 1991, Earvin "Magic" Johnson Jr. announced he was HIV positive. He retired from basketball to become one of the most prominent HIV/AIDS activists.

(continued from page 58)

as amfAR Countdown to a Cure for AIDS launched a research initiative in 2014 that aims to find scientific evidence for a cure. According to amfAR's website, the success of the "Berlin patient" in 2008 provided a blueprint for scientists to work with. The Berlin patient, also known as Timothy Brown, is the only known individual to be cured of HIV. There are said to be three factors that could have contributed to the success of the Berlin Patient. First, Brown was diagnosed with acute myeloid leukemia and underwent chemotherapy. According to Jon Cohen's article for ScienceMag.org:

The first is the process of conditioning, in which doctors destroyed Brown's own immune system with chemotherapy and whole body irradiation to prepare him for his bone marrow transplant ... He found a bone marrow donor who had a rare mutation in a gene that cripples a key receptor on white blood cells the virus uses to establish an infection ... The third possibility is his new immune system attacked remnants of his old one that held HIV-infected cells, a process known as graft versus host disease.

> There are still many unanswered questions, and doctors are working on a new plan of action in the next scientific phase to help uncover a cure for HIV.

your medication to ensure the bacteria is out of your system. Syphilis, gonorrhea, chlamydia, and trichomoniasis are STDs that can be easily treated with an antibiotic.

An STD might recur if your doctor prescribes you the wrong medication, or if you found antibiotics on your own and didn't choose the right medication. It is imperative that a health-care professional correctly identifies the infection to ensure they are providing you the correct antibiotics to treat the infection. STDs are not all created by the same pathogen, making them unique and requiring their own treatment plan.

If you fail to tell your regular sexual partner about the STD, it is possible that you can spread the infection back and forth. Telling your sexual partner allows them to seek treatment to prevent your risk of getting the infection again. When you have both

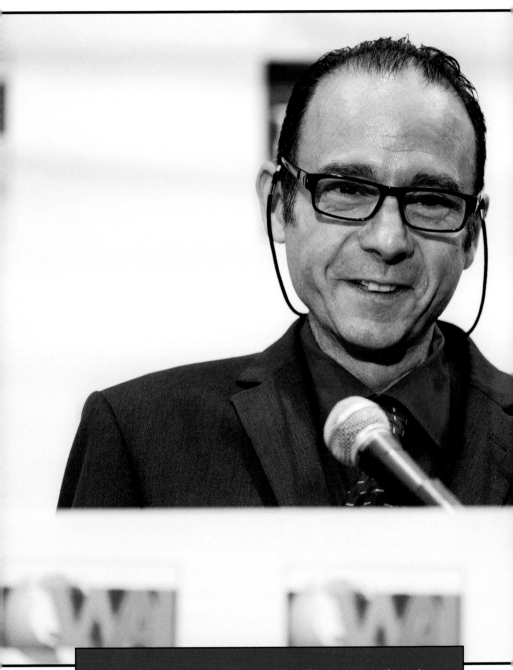

Timothy Ray Brown, the "Berlin patient," is known as the only person to be cured of HIV. He opened the Timothy Ray Brown Foundation to focus on finding a cure for the viral infection.

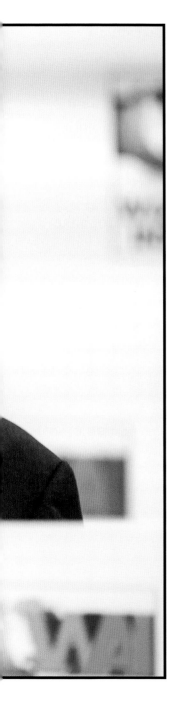

received treatment for the STD, you will have to wait a certain amount of time in order for the medication to run its course before returning to sexual activities—and most particularly, unprotected sexual contact. One of the main reasons that people get infected with STDs over and over again is because they continue to engage in unprotected sexual contact with partners who have untreated STDs. If you have been diagnosed with an STD and you do not want it to return, you may need to change your behavior to decrease the risk of contracting another STD. One of the smartest ways to prepare yourself is by always practicing safe sex and openly communicating with your partners about the risks.

For people who are diagnosed with chlamydia, it is possible for the infection to return. At first, doctors thought an encore of chlamydia was simply people being exposed to the infection again, but research has suggested that chlamydia can hide in your gut and reemerge at a later time.

Another STD that has been known to reemerge is gonorrhea. Gonorrhea has become antibiotic resistant and once commonly prescribed antibiotics can no longer effectively treat the infection. People who contract gonorrhea may need to be treated with expensive medication. After the treatment, it is suggested that the patient be tested again to make sure the treatment has worked.

Looking Ahead to a Bright Future

There are many ways to move forward with your life after a diagnosis, such as advocating for increased sex education at school or working with a community organization to help put an end to the stigma often associated with having an STD. You have an exciting future ahead of you, and your status does not define who you are and what you can accomplish. As retired professional basketball player Magic Johnson once said about his HIV-positive status, "HIV changed my life, but it doesn't keep me from living."

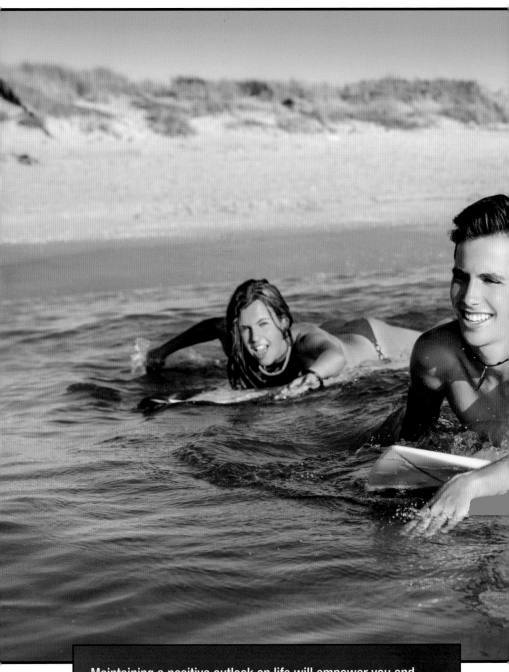

Maintaining a positive outlook on life will empower you and make you more confident. An STD diagnosis does not define who you are and what you can accomplish.

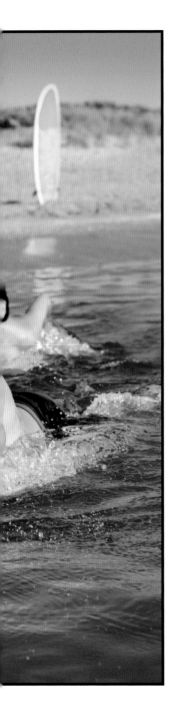

Understanding and Putting an End to the Stigma

Throughout history, many people have associated a positive STD diagnosis with "dirty" people. This is far from the truth. According to Jenelle Marie Pierce's article for the STD Project, "Another common metaphor surrounding genital herpes, as with many other STIs, is the idea that someone infected with HSV is 'dirty.'" The article explains that the metaphor has been around since the nineteenth century. It continues, "Specific diseases, such as cholera, as well as the state of being generally prone to illness, were thought to be caused by an 'infected' (or 'foul') atmosphere." Fast-forward to today, and there are still many negative stigmas associated with an STD diagnosis.

One of the most common stigmas associated with an STD

is that the person who has one is promiscuous. A major concern with that stigma is that it keeps people from getting tested, talking to their partners, and practicing safer sex. Risk isn't determined on the number of sexual partners you have because anyone can become infected if they are sexually active. There is always risk involved if there is sexual contact. Although we live in a highly sexualized society, people are interested in dictating another person's sex life, sometimes in a way that shames people. They are curious about who you are having sex with and how often. This type of sexual shaming is a way to scare people into having or not having sex. People are often put into the "naughty" category if they contract an STD. The fact is, though, that anyone can contract an STD, even people who have never had sexual intercourse or oral sex, or someone having sex for the first time. All different types of people

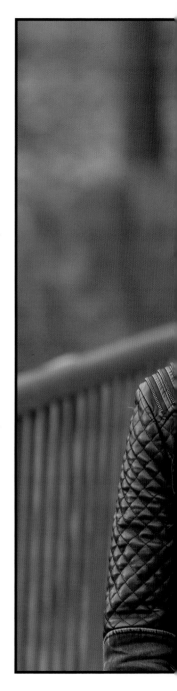

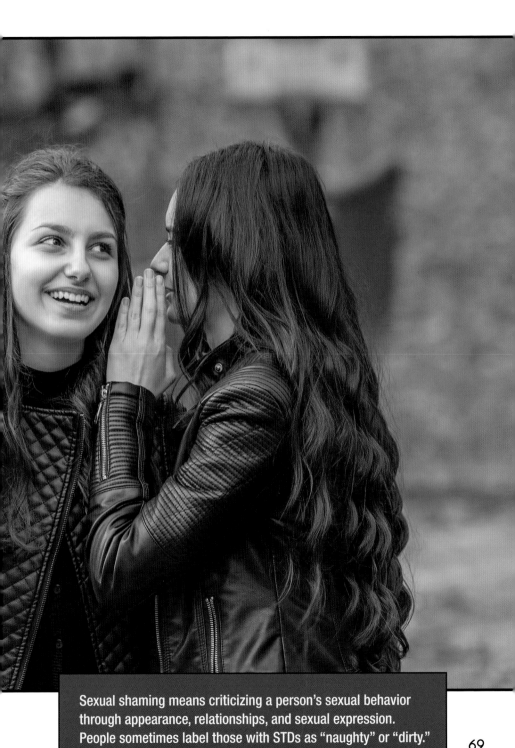

Sexual shaming means criticizing a person's sexual behavior through appearance, relationships, and sexual expression. People sometimes label those with STDs as "naughty" or "dirty."

from various backgrounds and ethnicities contract STDs all the time. Contracting an STD does not make you promiscuous or dirty.

Genital herpes is an STD that is often heard in many jokes. If you have seen the movie *The Hangover* (2009), you might remember the famous line, "What happens in Vegas, stays in Vegas. Except for herpes." This draws attention to the stigma surrounding herpes, which has been around for a long time, and no one knows where it originated. But the jokes are still often heard on television and in movies. If the statistics are correct, and one out of every four sexually active individuals has genital herpes, then a joke from a movie in a crowded theater might leave some people with hurt feelings.

To help end the stigma surrounding STDs, you need to support people with an STD. Try to imagine them in their own class like LGBTQ+ or people with disabilities and try to understand their struggle. Education is key to understanding STDs. Make sure to educate yourself and try to stop using metaphors when thinking about STDs. For example, people who have genital herpes are "unclean." Pay attention to common stereotypes regarding STDs, such as "she's a whore who probably has herpes," and correct people who say

How Effective Are Condoms?

Condoms are said to be the next best thing to abstinence in preventing the spread of an STD or preventing an unwanted pregnancy. They provide a barrier for any vaginal or penile secretions to be transmitted to your partner. While condoms won't protect you from an STD or pregnancy 100 percent of the time, they are the next best thing to abstinence. According to the World Health Organization, "When used correctly and consistently, condoms offer one of the most effective methods of protection against STIs, including HIV."

When using a condom, make sure to first check the expiration date on the condom. If the condom is expired, it might become dry and crack, which lets infections seep through. Latex condoms are known to be the most effective at preventing the spread of an STD, so when it comes time to choose the proper condom, latex might be the best decision. Keep in mind, however, that some people are allergic to latex. If you are allergic to latex, you can opt for a polyurethane condom instead.

(continued on the next page)

(continued from the previous page)

The most important thing to remember when using a condom to prevent the spread of STDs is using the condom correctly every time. Do not expose condoms to heat and light, which can dry out the condom and cause cracks. If you are using a lubricant in combination with a condom, make sure to find a water-based lubricant. Baby oil, lotion, and other types of lubricants can break down the condom and lead to condom breakage. If a condom accidentally slips off or breaks during sexual contact, you will need to contact your health-care provider and both parties will need to be tested for STDs—and pregnancy, if applicable.

such phrases. If everyone hides behind the stigma and lets the jokes continue, there will be no growth toward acceptance. Speak up if you hear any negative conversation or jokes about STDs. Your voice can make a difference. You can also tell your story anonymously if you feel more comfortable. The more you talk about it, the more empowered you will feel. Your efforts may also help others feel empowered to make a difference.

Be an Advocate for Change

If you want to educate people, help end the stigma associated with STDs, and advocate for STD prevention, there are many ways to jump in and make a difference.

ASHA Ambassadors

ASHA Ambassadors, through the American Sexual Health Association, are volunteers who share information regarding sexual and reproductive health via social media outlets. The Ambassadors use the social media platform to share updated and important information regarding sexual health. They are passionate about starting conversations that cover taboo topics in hopes of creating a nation that is sexually educated and healthy. Through the volunteer program, you can also find National Cervical Cancer Coalition (NCCC) chapters across the United States to help educate local communities about cervical cancer and HPV. ASHA Ambassadors are active in over twenty-six states. They also represent more than twenty countries across the globe. Being such a diverse group of people, everyone involved adds a unique perspective toward sexual and reproductive health.

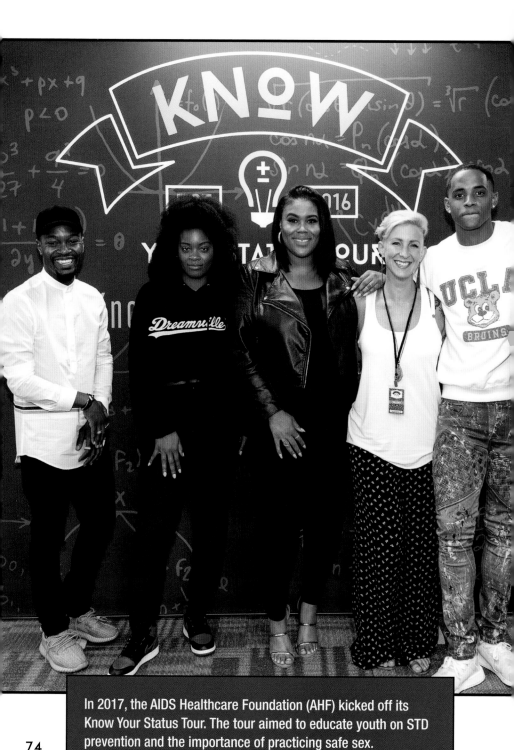

In 2017, the AIDS Healthcare Foundation (AHF) kicked off its Know Your Status Tour. The tour aimed to educate youth on STD prevention and the importance of practicing safe sex.

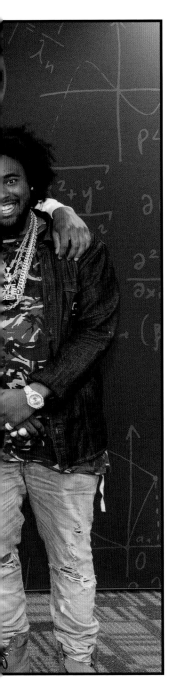

Advocates for Youth

Advocates for Youth's website, AdvocatesForYouth.org, helps youth find their voice. If you want your school to get more comprehensive sex education, increased information on STD and HIV testing, and condom availability, Advocates for Youth is a website you should explore. Its vision is to create a society that accepts sexuality as something that is natural and normal and incorporating young people as a resource. Engaging Communities Around HIV Organizing (ECHO) is an outreach program for young people who are HIV positive to help end the stigma toward HIV. ECHO leaders use social media, education, and media outreach to raise awareness about HIV and how it interconnects with homophobia, transphobia, and racism. One of their main goals is to educate communities about the impact HIV has on people of color, homosexuals, and the transgender community. Activists also participate in a storytelling campaign called My Story Out Loud, which gives a voice to LGBTQ+ youth across America.

Advocates for Youth also uses activists called student organizers, who are high school and college students who use their voice on a local and national level to spread the word about sexual rights for youth. They regularly campaign for the distribution of free menstrual products and condoms, the right for gender-neutral restrooms, and the right for access to comprehensive sexual education in schools, including HIV prevention and LGBTQ+ rights and health. Advocates for Youth offers many ways for young people to get involved in the fight for sexual health.

The STD Project

Sharing your story with a support group could also be beneficial and help you feel empowered. The STD Project website, TheSTDProject

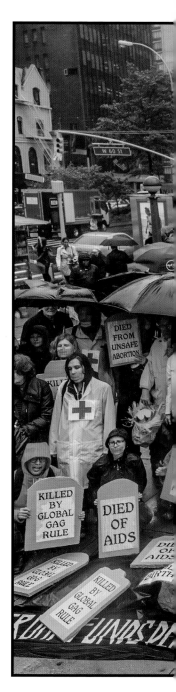

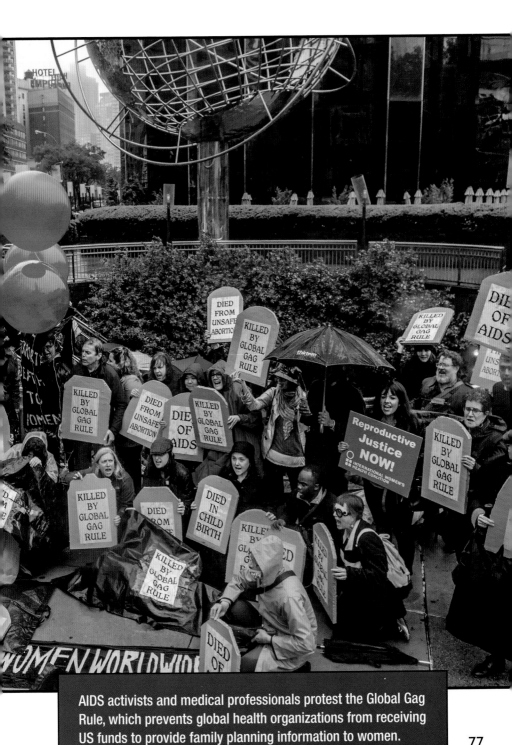

AIDS activists and medical professionals protest the Global Gag Rule, which prevents global health organizations from receiving US funds to provide family planning information to women.

.com, lists STD support groups by the type of STD, such as herpes, HPV, or HIV. Support groups for individuals who have been diagnosed with HPV and herpes are called HELP groups. The STD Project has a link that can connect you with a HELP group in your state, as well as contact information. Additionally, you can find HELP groups in Australia and Canada.

Depending on the location of the HELP group, you can find online support forums or an in-person meeting. The organization also lists support groups by location for HIV, including Canadian support groups and even worldwide support groups. If you do not see a support group of interest, the STD Project encourages you to reach out so it can better direct you toward a support group that best fits your needs.

Through the STD Project, you can also share your story with others anonymously. On the STD Project's website, there is a questionnaire that you can fill out in the form of an interview. It asks questions such as, "What type of STD do you have/had?," "How has your life changed since you contracted an STD?," and "How old are you?" It allows you to have the power to share as much or as little as you feel comfortable.

The STD Project also has a questionnaire for people who have been impacted by a friend or family member who was diagnosed with an STD.

This interview is called the People Who Love People with STIs Interview. After the submission of your interview, you will be contacted via email to let you know your submission has been received. The website advises the following: "Please remember to be patient with our publishing process depending on what's happening behind the scenes, sometimes it takes a little while for us to schedule your submission. But rest assured, we will definitely include your story."

CHAPTER SIX

Additional Resources at Your Fingertips

There are many resources to further educate yourself on STDs, testing, and prevention. The rise of the digital age has made it easier to access information regarding sexual health, but sometimes that is not enough. STD education and prevention should start at home and in schools. In the United States, however, not everyone is on board with comprehensive sexual education, and many schools still teach abstinence only. The rise of STDs among young people, most particularly people aged fifteen to twenty-five, suggest that abstinence-only programs are not effective at stopping teenagers from having sex. On its website, STDCheck states, "In some states, sex education cannot be taught unless it stresses abstinence before marriage. A bill proposed in one of those states, Utah, to allow parents to opt-in to comprehensive sex ed for their children was killed."

Today, sex should be taught as something that is normal and healthy, and not something that should induce shame or guilt. Over the past few years, there has been a rise in YouTube videos for young people who want to learn about sex education. Dr. Lindsey Doe, a sex educator, started a YouTube channel called Sexplanations, where she teaches people about masturbation and oral sex. The way in which Doe delivers her educational videos helps neutralize the subject matter, such as wearing a funny costume in combination with neutral facial expressions. She helps her audience feel comfortable while she delivers her sexual education lesson. There is also a channel called Queer Kid Stuff for younger people to learn about gender identity and sexuality. Host Lindsay Amer, along with her friend Teddy, discuss topics such as homophobia and diversity. The channel's LGBTQ+ videos aim to teach kids what is means to be LGBTQ+, and its

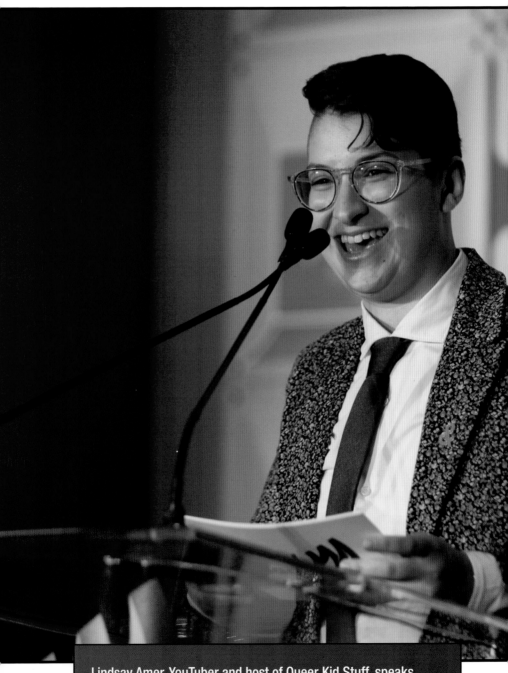

Lindsay Amer, YouTuber and host of Queer Kid Stuff, speaks during a 2017 GLAAD gala. The event celebrated the acceptance of LGBTQ+ people through digital influence.

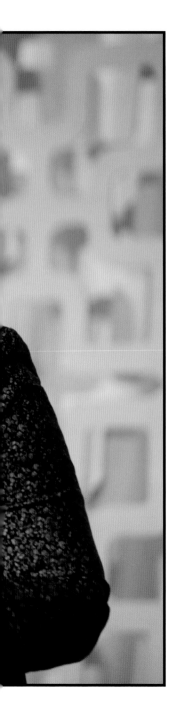

educational videos explain what the concepts of transgender and gender identity mean in theory and practicality.

The STD Project

For additional information regarding STD testing, personal stories, and STD stigma, the STD Project is a robust, award-winning website that caters to all things related to STDs. Jenelle Marie Pierce founded the site in 2012. Pierce serves as the spokesperson for Positive Singles, a dating website dedicated to people with STDs, and she is the founder of Herpes Activists Networking to Dismantle Stigma (HANDS). Pierce was diagnosed with genital herpes when she was sixteen years old and now dedicates her time to ending the stigma and opening up the conversation for STDs. In a personal statement on the STD Project website, Pierce states, "I understand what it's like to feel

Offering Helping HANDS

Herpes Activists Networking to Dismantle Stigma (HANDS) is an extension of the STD Project that gives readers information on the herpes virus. Its vision is to end the stigma toward herpes and make it more comfortable to open the conversation around herpes. HANDS also aims to empower people who have been diagnosed with herpes to enhance their sexual and physical health. The group believes that sexual health enables you to live a healthy life with a healthy body and mindset, you are allowed to have a fulfilling sex life and healthy relationships, and you are allowed to have peace of mind toward your diagnosis.

(continued on page 86)

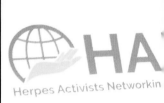

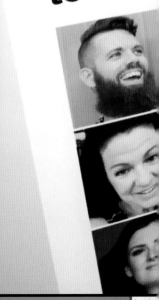

S

Stigma

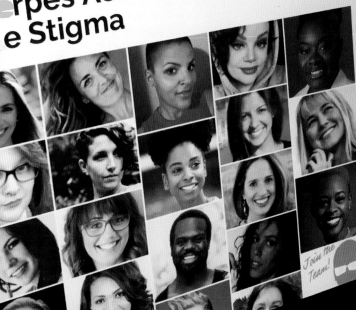

PTH   PERSPECTIVES   PREVENTION   **RESOURCES**

rpes Activists Networking
e Stigma

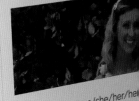

Jenelle Marie Pierce (she/her/her
Executive Director of Herpes.Educ
The STD Project; the Founder of th
activists network, HANDS; the
Spokesperson for Positive Singles
Tri-Chair of the Communications
Group at the National Coalition fo
Health (NCSH). She is also proof a
not a deal-breaker or the end of y
– rather, it is merely an unexpecte
ball in this interesting game we c
Learn more about her story on h
page, or find her socially below

Join the
Team!

Members of HANDS, an extension of the STD Project, promote
the acceptance of and education about herpes in hopes of
eradicating the negative stigma associated with the STD.

(continued from page 84)

To become a member of HANDS, you must agree with the overall values and goals that HANDS stands for, but you do not have to agree with what every member is doing in their HANDS endeavor. There are two membership options for anyone who is interested in joining HANDS. Both memberships include conference calls every quarter and participation in every project. Public membership will allow you to be listed in the member directory. It also allows you to have full voting rights, where as an associate membership is not listed in the member directory and you do not have permission to vote. The HANDS team works together to uplift everyone's individual endeavors and provides the community with up-to-date information and accurate resources for the herpes virus.

stereotyped, misunderstood, and alone with something considered taboo. As a result, I work to encourage education and facilitate thoughtful discussion about sexual health and STDs."

The STD Project has an abundance of information for people who are facing the diagnosis of an STD. On its website, it breaks down the different STDs into categories, such as viral STDs, bacterial STDs, and parasitic STDs. There is also a section for additional support, which includes books and how to find a private STD testing center that provides fast results that is also affordable. The award-winning website has been featured in the *New York Times*, on CBS News, on CNN, and in *Forbes*. It has also received many awards, such as the Top 40 Sexual Health Blogs and Websites on March 15, 2018, and the Top 100 Sex Blogging Superheroes on October 31, 2017. If you are wondering where to start, the STD Project is a great place to gain wonderful information and education on everything related to STDs.

Planned Parenthood

A great resource for STD information is your local Planned Parenthood. Planned Parenthood offers information regarding sexual health education, STD testing and treatment, and planning your visit to the doctor. A wealth of information is available at Planned Parenthood, and a lot of the resources can be found online without having to walk into a clinic. On its website, Planned Parenthood lists itself as a top provider of quality health care and sex education. Most of the services it offers are covered for free and without a co-payment. These include birth control, HIV testing, and STD testing. Planned

Parenthood does not accept walk-in appointments, so you must make an appointment to be seen. If you are uncomfortable talking on the phone, you have the option to privately book an appointment via their online portal.

Educator and nurse Margaret Sanger founded Planned Parenthood on October 16, 1916. Sanger believed that women should be in control of their bodies and their futures. In 1923, Sanger distributed birth control devices and collected information regarding long-term use of birth control when she opened the Birth Control Clinical Research Bureau in Manhattan, New York. Her forward-thinking approach jump-started a movement, and in 1936, it was ruled that birth control could be legally obtained in New York, Vermont, and Connecticut. Birth control was no longer labeled as indecent. PlannedParenthood .org notes the following: "While it took another 30 years for these

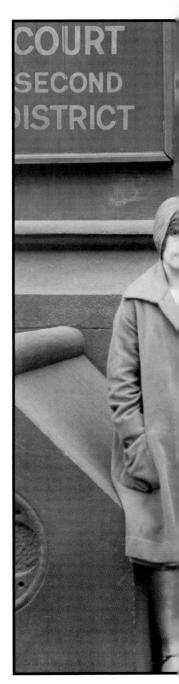

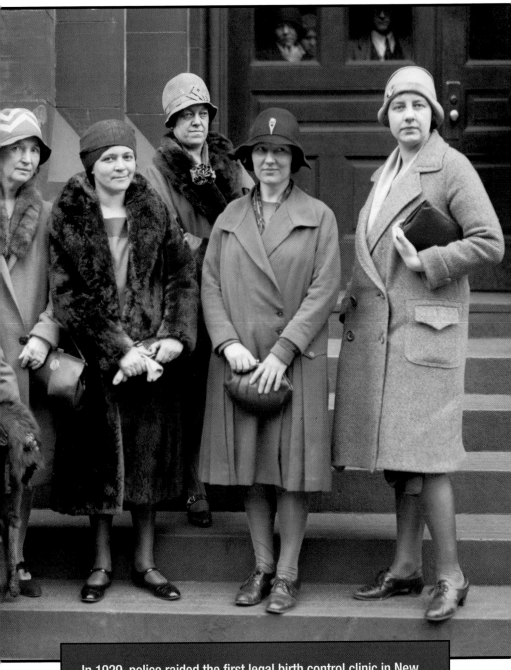

In 1929, police raided the first legal birth control clinic in New York—opened by Margaret Sanger in 1923—and arrested a doctor and staff members. Charges were later dropped.

rights to be extended to married couples (but just married couples) throughout the rest of the country, it was an historic step toward making birth control available to everyone." In 2011, Planned Parenthood went global to provide sexual health and reproductive information and care to twelve countries. The website states, "More than 4.3 million people have received sexual and reproductive health information and services provided by partners, including more than 2 million adolescents and youth."

The Planned Parenthood website is easy to navigate. On the main page, it has a section called "For Teens" that gives young people information on sex, relationships, preventing STDs and pregnancy, and much more. While navigating through the different subjects on the website, a chat option will pop up called Roo. Roo allows you to ask confidential questions about sex and STDs, and even pose questions about your body. Roo will never ask for your personal information, so you can be assured that all questions asked are private and kept confidential. Roo can help you get answers to any question that you may find too embarrassing to ask an adult. All of Roo's answers are backed by Planned Parenthood's sexual health experts, so you can feel confident that the information you receive is accurate.

American Sexual Health Association (ASHA)

ASHA was founded in 1914 during the height of early twentieth-century social reforms. The organization was focused mainly on fighting STDs, but back in 1914, STDs were called venereal diseases (VD). The mission of ASHA is promoting the sexual health of the public through education to foster healthy sexual behaviors. Its website states, "The American Sexual Health Association (ASHA) envisions a world where sexual and reproductive health and rights are universally recognized, and where comprehensive sexual health information and services are accessible and available to all."

The ASHA website, ASHASexualHealth.org, offers a service where a person can ask a question to a doctor regarding their sexual health or STD for a fee called Ask the Experts. The benefit of Ask the Experts is that you can ask a question on your own time without leaving the comfort of your home. There is an option to browse a series of questions that have already been answered by a team of health-care professionals. If you do not see a question you would like to ask, ASHA charges $25 per question and offers up to two follow-up questions without further charge. If you don't want to wait for an

HOW TO PRACTICE
SAFE SEX
SEXUALLY TRANSMITTED DISEASES PREVENTION

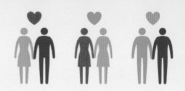

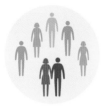

**LIMIT THE NUMBER
OF PARTNERS**

**AVOID ALCOHOL
AND DRUG ABUSE**

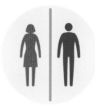

PRACTICE ABSTINENCE

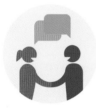

**TALK OPENLY
WITH YOUR PARTNER**

**GET TESTED TO KNOW
IF YOU HAVE STD**

**GET MEDICAL TREATMENT
TO PREVENT OR CURE STD**

**WASH BEFORE AND AFTER
SEXUAL INTERCOURSE**

**USE A LATEX OR
POLYURETHANE CONDOM**

**USE PROTECTION
FOR ALL FORMS OF SEX**

The prevention of STDs starts with education on practicing safe sex. Taking precautions can greatly minimize a person's risk of spreading or contracting an STD.

answer you can utilize the Person2Person option. The Person2Person option allows you to speak with a staff member to get a question answered through online chat or by telephone. Through this paid service, you can decide when you want to talk to someone and for how long, putting you in charge of your sexual health.

A popular slogan on its website is "Yes Means Test." If you are responsible and mature enough to engage in sexual intercourse, you should be mature enough to get tested for STDs. There is an option to find an STD testing center that will give the reader more information on the nearest clinic. Entering your zip code will create a list of testing sites nearby with helpful information on cost and the types of testing they provide. Many, if not all, of the clinics offer HIV testing free of charge.

Although STDs are on the rise in the United States and globally, there are many beneficial resources available to educate yourself and get tested if you are sexually active. The world is changing to make resources readily available with the click of a mouse. There are many support groups, blogs, and confidential online question forums to open the conversation about sexual health and STDs. The hard work of organizations such as Planned Parenthood, the American Sexual Health Association, and the STD Project are normalizing education on STDs to

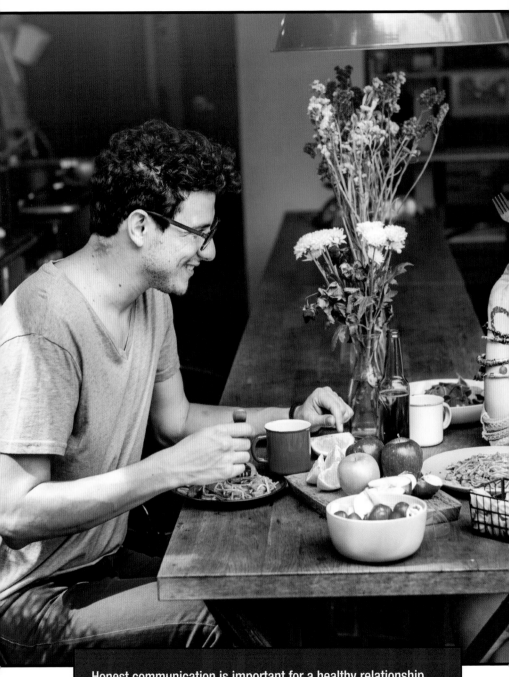

Honest communication is important for a healthy relationship. Being an active listener and talking openly with your partner will bring you closer, build trust, and boost mutual respect.

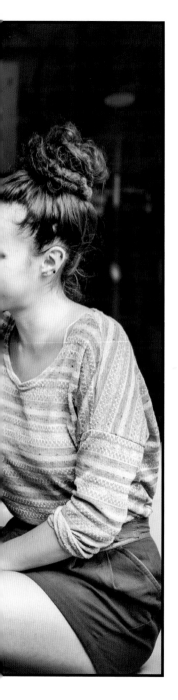

create a future where STDs aren't taboo. Also, amfAR is leading the way in its research to finding a cure for HIV by the end of 2020.

One day, we can all envision a world where STDs are treated as something that is normal. The most important thing you can do if you are sexually active or thinking of becoming sexually active is to educate yourself and get tested. Respect yourself and your body, as well as your sexual partners, and make STD testing a priority.

Glossary

abstinence The personal decision to not engage in sexual activities or sexual intercourse.

antibiotics Prescription medication that fights infections caused by bacteria.

birth control The active use of contraception to prevent an unwanted or accidental pregnancy.

chemotherapy A type of cancer treatment that aims to shrink tumors, prolong life, and destroy cancer cells in the body.

cognitive behavioral therapy (CBT) A goal-oriented form of talk therapy that is short-term and targets negative thoughts and behavior.

condom A thin layer of material that creates a barrier to prevent the spread of STDs and prevent pregnancy.

confidential A verbal or written act of secrecy, often for the protection of the patient.

dental dam A thin piece of latex that is worn over a person's genitals or anus to prevent the spread of STDs through mouth-to-genital or mouth-to-anus interaction.

discriminate To make an assumption about someone based on a person's group, category, race, or class.

epidemiologist A medical expert in the distribution and control of diseases.

gender identity A person's internal sense and identification of the sex they were born or something different. It is decided by how the person sees themself.

guardian A person who is legally accountable for the management and well-being of a minor.

heterosexual A person who is sexually attracted to a member of the opposite sex.

homophobia Negative feelings or hatred toward homosexuality.

infertility The inability to produce children.

LGBTQ+ An acronym for lesbian, gay, bisexual, transgender, queer (or questioning), pansexual, asexual, nonbinary, and gender variant.

over-the-counter A term used to describe medications that can be purchased at a pharmacy or drug store without a prescription.

sexting The act of sending and receiving sexually explicit text messages.

stereotype A generalized belief or idea about a group of people.

stigma The discrimination or disapproval of someone's characteristics or situation.

support system A group or network of people who support the emotional and mental health of another person.

symptom A physical or mental characteristic that is produced from a mental or physical condition or issue.

taboo Referring to a social custom that is not often talked about in mainstream society.

tattoo A permanent mark made on an individual's body by inserting ink or dye into the skin with a needle.

transgender An adjective used to describe a person's gender expression or identity that does not match their assigned gender at birth.

venereal disease (VD) A term used in the early twentieth century to describe an infection or disease caused by sexual contact.

virus A microorganism that can cause an infection by replicating itself while inside a living host.

Action Canada for Sexual Health and Rights

251 Bank Street, 2nd Floor

Ottawa, ON K2P1X3

Canada

(888) 642-2725

Website: http://www.actioncanadaSHR.org

Email: info@actioncanadashr.org

Facebook: @actioncanadaSHR

Twitter: @actioncanadashr

YouTube: Action Canada for Sexual Health and Rights

Action Canada for Sexual Health and Rights works with decision makers to promote sexual education, gender equality, and LGBTQ+ rights.

American Sexual Health Association (ASHA)

PO Box 13827

Durham, NC 27709

(919) 361-8400

Website: http://www.ashasexualhealth.org

Email: info@ashasexualhealth.org

Facebook: @americansexualhealthassociation

Twitter: @InfoASHA

YouTube: American Sexual Health Association

ASHA works to create a society where sexual health is recognized and information and services are readily available to individuals, families, and communities.

CATIE

555 Richmond Street West

Suite 505, Box 1104

Toronto, ON M5V 3B1

Canada

(416) 203-7122 or (800) 263-1638

Website: https://www.catie.ca

Email: info@catie.ca

Facebook and Twitter: @CATIEinfo

YouTube: CATIEinfo

CATIE creates accessible information for hepatitis C and HIV treatment, testing, and support to improve the health of all Canadians.

Foundation for AIDS Research (amfAR)

120 Wall Street, 13th Floor

New York, NY 10005-3908

(212) 806-1600

Website: https://www.amfAR.org

Email: info@amfar.org

Facebook: @amfarthefoundationforaidsresearch

Instagram: @amfar

Twitter: @amfAR

YouTube: amfAR :: The Foundation for AIDS Research

Founded in 2014, amfAR works to find scientific evidence to achieve a cure for HIV/AIDS or HIV remission by the end of 2020.

National Coalition for Sexual Health (NCSH)

(202) 375-7805

Website: https://www.nationalcoalitionforsexualhealth.org

Email: ncsh@altarum.org

Facebook: @NCSH2012

Twitter: NCSH_

NCSH promotes access to sexual health resources and encourages open communication about sexual health and education between families, partners, and communities.

Options for Sexual Health (Options)

3550 East Hastings Street

Vancouver, BC V5K 2A7

Canada

(800) 739-7367

Website: https://www.optionsforsexualhealth.org

Email: info@optionsforsexualhealth.org

Facebook and Twitter: @optbc

Since 1968, Options has promoted accessible sexual health education and health care for all. It offers reproductive health care and sexual health care services in the Yukon and British Columbia.

Planned Parenthood

(800) 230-PLAN

Website: https://www.plannedparenthood.org

Facebook: @PlannedParenthood

Instagram: @plannedparenthood

Twitter: @PPFA

YouTube: Planned Parenthood

Planned Parenthood provides quality health care and sexual health care at an affordable price in the United States and around the world. It specializes in STD treatment and testing, sexual education, birth control, and general health care.

Project Inform

25 Taylor Street, 7th Floor

San Francisco, CA 94102

(415) 558-8669

Website: https://www.projectinform.org

Email: support@projectinform.org

Facebook and Twitter: @ProjectInform

Instagram: @projectinform

Project Inform works to create a society that is free from HIV and hepatitis C by focusing on the development of drugs, education, prevention, and access to health care.

Scarleteen

5315 N. Clark Street #126

Chicago, IL 60640

(206) 866-2279

Website: http://www.scarleteen.com

Facebook and Twitter: @Scarleteen

Founded in 1998, Scarleteen is dedicated to providing up-to-date information on sexual health and relationships. Scarleteen also provides interactive services, including message boards, live chat and text/SMS services, referrals for STD testing, LGBTQ+ support, and crisis care.

The Trevor Project

PO Box 69232

West Hollywood, CA 90069

(866) 488-7386

Website: https://www.thetrevorproject.org

Email: info@thetrevorproject.org

Facebook: @TheTrevorProject

Instagram: @trevorproject

Twitter: @TrevorProject

YouTube: The Trevor Project

The Trevor Project was founded in 1988 and provides suicide prevention and crisis intervention for LGBTQ+ youth. It has a suicide hotline that is open twenty-four hours a day, seven days a week, for anyone who is suicidal and needs help.

For Further Reading

Corinna, Heather. *S.E.X.* Boston, MA: De Capo Lifelong Books, 2016.

Forna, Fatu. *From Your Doctor to You: What Every Teenage Girl Should Know About Her Body, Sex, STDs and Contraception.* Scotts Valley, CA: CreateSpace Independent Publishing Platform, 2014.

Freedman, Jeri. *Herpes* (Your Sexual Health). New York, NY: Rosen Young Adult, 2015.

Furgang, Kathy. *HIV/AIDS* (Your Sexual Health). New York, NY: Rosen Young Adult, 2015.

Grimes, Jill. *Seductive Decisions: How Everyday People Catch STIs.* Baltimore, MD: Johns Hopkins University Press, 2016.

Orr, Tamra. *Gonorrhea* (Your Sexual Health). New York, NY: Rosen Young Adult, 2015.

Staley, Erin. *HPV and Genital Warts.* New York, NY: Rosen Young Adult, 2015.

Vernacchio, Al. *For Goodness Sex: Changing the Way We Talk to Teens About Sexuality, Values, and Health.* New York, NY: Harper Wave, 2014.

Wolny, Philip. *I Have An STD. Now What?* New York, NY: Rosen Young Adult, 2015.

Wolny, Philip. *Syphilis* (Your Sexual Health). New York, NY: Rosen Young Adult, 2015.

Bibliography

American Cancer Society medical and editorial content team. "HPV Vaccines." American Cancer Society, October 8, 2018. https://www.cancer.org/cancer/cancer-causes /infectious-agents/hpv/hpv-vaccines.html.

Battaglia, Emily. "STD Facts: 10 Things You Need to Know." Everyday Health, September 24, 2018. https://www .everydayhealth.com/sexual-health/std-facts-10-things -you-need-know.

Boskey, Elizabeth. "Top 10 Reasons to Support Sex Education in Schools." Verywell Health, January 14, 2019. https:// www.verywellhealth.com/support-comprehensive -education-schools-3133083.

Cancer.org. "HPV and HPV Testing." February 18, 2019. https://www.cancer.org/cancer/cancer-causes/infectious -agents/hpv/hpv-and-hpv-testing.html.

Centers for Disease Control and Prevention. "Basic Statistics." Retrieved April 13, 2019. https://www.cdc.gov/hiv /basics/statistics.html.

Clark-Flory, Tracy. "So You Have an STD. Now What?" *Elle*, May 15, 2015. https://www.elle.com/life-love/sex -relationships/advice/a28391/std-notification-etiquette.

Cohen, Jon. "How Did the 'Berlin Patient' Rid Himself of HIV?" *Science*, September 25, 2014. https://www.sciencemag .org/news/2014/09/how-did-berlin-patient-rid-himself -hiv.

Dallas, Mary Elizabeth. "Behavioral Counseling Urged for Teens, Young Adults at Risk for STDs." Consumer HealthDay, September 22, 2014. https://consumer .healthday.com/general-health-information-16/doctor -news-206/behavioral-counseling-urged-for-teens -young-adults-at-risk-for-stds-691925.html.

Ethier, Kathleen, Laura Kann, and Timothy McManus. "Sexual Intercourse Among High School Students — 29 States and United States Overall, 2005–2015." Centers for Disease Control and Prevention (CDC), January 5, 2018. https://www.cdc.gov/mmwr/volumes/66/wr/mm665152a1.htm.

FDA News Release. "FDA Approves Expanded Use of Gardasil 9 to Include Individuals 27 Through 45 Years Old." US Food and Drug Administration (FDA), October 5, 2018. https://www.fda.gov/newsevents/newsroom/pressannouncements/ucm622715.htm.

Martin, Ben. "Challenging Negative Self Talk." PsychCentral, October 8, 2018. https://psychcentral.com/lib/challenging-negative-self-talk.

Morse, Emily. "What to Expect After an STI." Verywell Health, August 3, 2018. https://www.verywellhealth.com/what-to-expect-after-an-std-4082998.

Office of Adolescent Health. "Adolescent Development and STDs." HHS.gov: Office of Adolescent Health, US Department of Health & Human Services, September 12, 2016. https://www.hhs.gov/ash/oah/adolescent-development/reproductive-health-and-teen-pregnancy/stds/index.html.

Planned Parenthood. "Half of All Teens Feel Uncomfortable Talking to Their Parents About Sex While Only 19 Percent of Parents Feel the Same, New Survey Shows." January 30, 2014. https://www.plannedparenthood.org/about-us/newsroom/press-releases/half-all-teens-feel-uncomfortable-talking-their-parents-about-sex-while-only-19-percent-parents.

Planned Parenthood. "Planned Parenthood 100 Years." Retrieved March 23, 2019. https://100years.plannedparenthood.org.

Quinn, Paul. *Sexually Transmitted Diseases: Your Questions Answered.* Santa Barbara, CA: Greenwood, an imprint of ABC-CLIO, LLC, 2018.

Sifferlin, Alexandra. "Here's Why Teen STDs Are Hitting All-Time Highs." *Time,* November 7, 2016. http://time.com/4558627/heres-why-teen-stds-are-hitting-all-time-highs.

STDAware blog. "STD Resource Center: Everything You Need to Know About STDs." https://www.stdaware.com/std-resource-center.

Thompson, Dennis. "STD Rates Continue to Climb in U.S." WebMD, August 28, 2018. https://www.webmd.com/sexual-conditions/news/20180828/std-rates-continue-to-climb-in-us#1.

Torgovnik, Jonathan. "Sexually Transmitted Infections (STIs)." World Health Organization. https://www.who.int/news-room/fact-sheets/detail/sexually-transmitted-infections-(stis).

White, Krishna Wood, MD. "HIV and AIDS." KidsHealth, October 2018. https://kidshealth.org/en/parents/hiv.html.

Woolsey, Barbara. "How Scientists Are Getting Closer to Wiping Out STDs." Thrillist, July 22, 2016. https://www.thrillist.com/sex-dating/nation/the-future-of-curable-stds.

Index

About the Author

Jacqueline Parrish graduated from Appalachian State University with a bachelor of arts in English literature. She was a freelance writer for a local publication while in college. Parrish dedicates her time to maintaining a healthy lifestyle and staying up to date on sexual health and education. In her free time, she enjoys reading, writing, book collecting, and barre class. She resides in Kalamazoo, Michigan, with her daughter, Madeline.

Photo Credits